YOUR KNOWLEDGE HAS VALUE

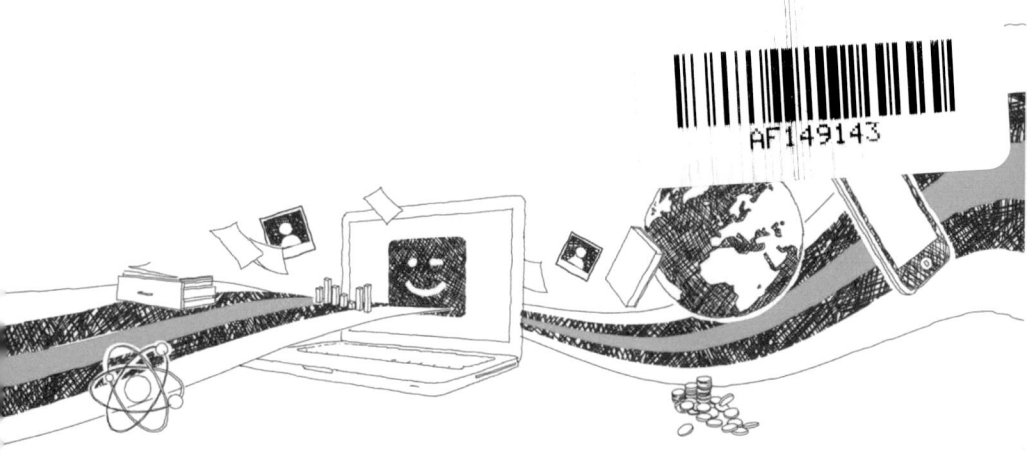

AF149143

- We will publish your bachelor's and master's thesis, essays and papers

- Your own eBook and book - sold worldwide in all relevant shops

- Earn money with each sale

Upload your text at www.GRIN.com
and publish for free

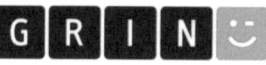

Bibliographic information published by the German National Library:

The German National Library lists this publication in the National Bibliography; detailed bibliographic data are available on the Internet at http://dnb.dnb.de .

This book is copyright material and must not be copied, reproduced, transferred, distributed, leased, licensed or publicly performed or used in any way except as specifically permitted in writing by the publishers, as allowed under the terms and conditions under which it was purchased or as strictly permitted by applicable copyright law. Any unauthorized distribution or use of this text may be a direct infringement of the author s and publisher s rights and those responsible may be liable in law accordingly.

Imprint:

Copyright © 2016 GRIN Verlag, Open Publishing GmbH
Print and binding: Books on Demand GmbH, Norderstedt Germany
ISBN: 9783668246041

This book at GRIN:

http://www.grin.com/en/e-book/334449/personalized-medicine-for-brain-disorders-new-hope-old-problems

Ekaterina Kopeikina

Personalized medicine for brain disorders. New hope, old problems

GRIN Publishing

GRIN - Your knowledge has value

Since its foundation in 1998, GRIN has specialized in publishing academic texts by students, college teachers and other academics as e-book and printed book. The website www.grin.com is an ideal platform for presenting term papers, final papers, scientific essays, dissertations and specialist books.

Visit us on the internet:

http://www.grin.com/

http://www.facebook.com/grincom

http://www.twitter.com/grin_com

PERSONALIZED MEDICINE OF BRAIN DISORDERS: NEW HOPE, OLD PROBLEMS

It is often said that 21st century is the century of neuroscience. With several moon-shot projects targeting the whole connectome of human brain, computer modelling of neural networks and mapping of brain functions using neuroimaging it might well be the case.

However, the situation in clinics remains a catastrophe. There is no effective treatment for most neurodegenerative and psychiatric diseases. And the development of new drugs is not progressing fast enough. With an increasing social and economic burden of neurological diseases, we face a sad disproportion in funds and resources provided by private pharmacological companies and government projects targeting the brain diseases in comparison to cancer, vascular diseases and viral infections. Those drugs that are currently prescribed were developed in mid-20th century with all the derivatives to be basically the same [1].

Cutting-edge fields like personalized genomics is one of the potential game-changing solutions for boosting the neurological and psychiatric treatment. Still, its usage has its own limitations. Let us consider both possibilities and complications of this approach.

1. PROS

1.1 LESS BIAS AND FOCUS ON HUMAN

Common clinical research is based on the hypothesis validation, which means a researcher must come up with a possible cause based on clinical and experimental evidence and even beforehand. The other way to find a new treatment is serendipity when new or old chemical substance being reported to alleviate some symptoms just by a pure chance. However, with advanced data mining and machine learning algorithms bioinformatics can screen the databases of patients for the common genes and SNPs even without the pathways of interest. That can provide a deeper understanding of the complex mechanism of disease and reveal new unintuitive targets.

Genome-vide studies or discovery of rare genetic variants are already helping to discover common mechanisms and pathways of such seemingly unrelated conditions as Alzheimer's and Parkinson's diseases, autism, eating disorders, epilepsy, schizophrenia, and major depression[2].

Another major advantage is using human clinic data. It is often the case that the newly developed treatment shows promising results on animals, but there are difficulty in translation this success on stage III and IV of clinical trials. The reason is poor model of the disease, and with the complex and evolutionary late cognitive and memory processes it is almost impossible to repeat the exact disorder in animal models.

1.2 STATISTICAL POWER

The sample size is both a strength and weakness of individual genomics. Most of the samples of neurological studies are small, with 100 patients or less. When it comes to rare mutations the number can start from only the single case.

However, the collaboration of research groups across the institutions and online data-bases of genomes allow to reach large-scale samples exceeding 100,000 individuals

Such comprehensive meta-analysis already provides new insights on schizophrenia, Alzheimer's, epilepsy, multiple sclerosis, bipolar illness, major depression, and ADHD, autism, anorexia nervosa, recovery after stroke, and Parkinson's disease. Just as an example, more than 100 genetic loci in risk for the epilepsy have been found.

Finally, the emphasis on human allows to compare independent cohorts with numerous factors having a huge impact on treatment progression. One of the examples in neurology is a screening for the HLA-B*1502 allele in Asian patients which helped to prevent seizures onset during the clinical trials. Such factors as gender, age and ethnicity often plays an important role when it comes to drug response, with different groups benefited or had severe-side effects on the same treatment[3].

1.3 INDIVIDUAL DRUG RESPONSE

So, personalized genomics can be applied on every step of treatment, from initial choose of an appropriate to observing the patient response to it. The patient response on the same drug differs dramatically. It has been long known in clinics, including psychopharmacology. On clinical trial phase II it is important to finally determine which group of patients will be resistant or sensitive to the drug and establish effective but least toxic dosage for them.

In the 1970s it has been observed that debrisoquine caused a different response, dividing patients into two distinct groups of its metabolism. It was explained later by different cytochrome P450 (CYP) 2D6 enzyme activity. Nowadays, 84% of known antidepressants have CYP2D6 and CYP2C19 metabolizer status labeling and the Polymorphisms in the CYP2D6 gene (rs1065852 and rs1080985) are associated with donepezil efficacy in Alzheimer's cognitive impairment alleviation. Also pharmacogenomic test for these genes have been approved[4].

Individual genomics can help to ease and increase the speed in differentiating the states with common symptoms and different etiology, like epilepsy. epilepsy suggesting ketogenic diet in glucose transporter type 1 deficiency syndrome or not prescribing lamotrigine, phenytoin, and carbamazepine in Dravet syndrome[4].

In 2014 the Table of Pharmacogenomic Biomarkers used by FDA in USA listed 145 precautions for 24 psychiatry prescriptions, 9 neurology treatments and 2 anesthetic drugs. And these list is expected to constantly expand. For example, a polymorphism in the gene OCT1/SLC22A1 affect the effectiveness of anti-Parkinsonian drugs[3].

1.4 TARGETED THERAPY

Not only the drug response screening, but the gene targeted treatment is an ultimate goal of personalized genomics.

With the discovery in 1989 single mutation responsible for cystic fibrosis, there was a hope that we will map all the genes connected to all known diseases. Due to complex gene-gene and gene-environment interactions, it might never be the case with brain-related illnesses. Yet, the patients with neurogenetic disorders such as Fragile X, Williams syndrome, and Turner syndrome, and partially Rett Syndrome and autism can already benefit from the personalized medicine approach due to the newly discovered genetic correlations[3].

For every case, obviously, the knowledge about the gene-phenotype connection is required. And that is a major field of research right now, with new computational methods developed. Some of the strongly correlated with the disease risk loci have already been established.

For Alzheimer's disease the mutations APP, PSEN1, and PSEN2 contribute to age and severity of the disease onset. The TOMMORROW trial is a phase III trial examining the TOMM40 genotypes. Variants of the glucocorticoid receptor gene NR3C1 contribute to schizophrenia and bipolar disorder. BDNF variants are linked with depression, Parkinson's and Alzheimer's disease[5].

As soon as the risk genes are found, gene therapy with adeno-associated virus (AAV) can be used as a more targeted way of using genomics and epigenomics in personalized medicine.

Epigenetic approach such as gene silencing by using vivo-Morpholinos and antisense oligonucleotides is also promising in the precision medicine[6].

The longitudinal studies are still needed to finally establish the weight of SNPs, gene and chromosome mutations on the susceptibility to the disease.

1.5 PREDICTION AND PREVENTION

A huge gain of personalized genomics is not even the treatment. It is prevention.

Even though now it is more of a possibility, than an established practice, already one can already take advantage of two usage of genome sequencing.

Firstly, you can estimate your own risk of the disease, and make choices accordingly, e.g. change your diet and lifestyle. Nutriegenomics, a whole new field of research in nature-nuture interconnection, could provide a scientific base for individually based diet for neurological disorders treatment and prophylactics.

Secondly, the parent can opt for in vitro fertilization to scan for genetically healthy embryos. With CRISPR/CAS9 and TALENs technology we can even adjust the genome of the cell, but right now the embryonic modification for actual pregnancy is generally prohibited. Chinese research groups have started and British have received permission to do embryo modification for research purposes.

Thus, a knowledge of individual variances can also help to avoid severe toxicity, estimate a right dosage and even predict drug resistance. And a final approval of the prescribed therapy is more often cannot be obtained without the risk gene screening.

2. CONS

2.1 PRACTICAL ISSUES

Event with state-of-the-art technologies as next-generation sequencing and CHIPs the whole-genome analysis is still far from being a universal clinical practice. One of the major reasons for that is its cost. Since the whole procedure is labor, time and knowledge demanding the estimated price for single patient in thousands of US dollars.

The other difficulty particularly neurological disorders is the access to brain of living patients due to the the skull and blood-brain barrier.

To obtain a genome database and interpret its meaning researches need data from not only current patients, but also healthy controls. Since whole gene sequencing becomes more wide spread there are different new concerns emerging. Insurance companies can already deny a support based on whether a patient has high risk of particular disease. New 'genome hackers' anxiety about scares people from doing a test due to insufficient anonymity and personal data security. And often government policy does not help either.

And also there is a high falsehood possibility. With modern technology it is possible not only to scan for target genes, but to use whole genome, exome and transcriptome sequencing. However, the data analysis, as actually the case with all clinical and scientific studies, is still a mix of objective and subjective interpretation. So, final conclusion and recommendations can be biased due to insufficient information about the gene or outrage fraud.

With all that said, there is a legal matter considering the patents for such treatment. Will the companies obscure the sequences or will they be for public usage? However ridiculous it might seem to own a gene, this might be the case.

2.2 SYSTEM RIGIDITY

Another issue to address is that current public healthcare system is mostly unsuitable for individual approach. It is one thing to show high efficacy for animal and human subjects in genetic research, another — to get a therapy approval from high authorities. Starting from impossibility of universal protocols to smaller samples in trials, personalized medicine struggles with conventional clinical trials regulations. Approving protocols for the gathering, analyzing and interpreting DNA data from human participants, along with education of clinicians in genetics counselling is a long bureaucratic process.

And even after the therapy is approved, you need physicians, molecular biologists and bioinformatics work together, which is not always the case in existent reality.

2.3 COMPLEXITY

To target revealed polymorphisms and genes we must be sure of their function. Most of the brain disorders are complex diseases which means that there is no single gene mutation leading to a disease.

Molecular pathways and structural patterns related to psychiatric disorders are still vague.

There are pathways, like mTOR dysregulation leads to various severe pathologies, from cancer to psychiatric syndromes. The down-regulation of this pathway, e.g. mTOR inhibition can be beneficial for dealing with symptoms of these diseases[7]. At the same time, for other cases, like depression treatment and immune stimulation, up-regulation is needed. So, tinkering with such complex genes in both directions we are facing the risk of severe side-effects.

The cell and tissue levels also fluctuate. Different neuronal subtypes have different features including receptors, excitability, structural and electrophysiological characteristics. With so many individual variances, it is often hard to define a phenotype of health and disease.

Mental health problems also lack of standard definitions. Weight loss and weight gain, sleep loss and excessive sleepiness can be both described as a depression symptoms, just to name a few.

2.3.1 ENVIRONMENT AND EPIGENETICS

Even with absolutely the same genotype there is a discordance within monozygotic twins. For example, DNA methylation CACNA1C, IGF2 and the p38 MAP kinase MAPK11 involved in glucocorticoid signaling lead to differences in depression onset possibility[8].

Epigenome modifies gene expression in response to environment changes. Lifestyle has a major impact on the epigenome. It includes nutrition, stress, physical activity and other environmental and social factors. Thus, simply to look for the gene correlation in complex neurological conditions is not enough.

It is important to find environmental and internal factors that actually cause the disease. Since the best way to treat the illness is to prevent it.

2.3.2 ETHICS AND SAFETY CONCERNS

Even when we find genes or SNPs responsible for the disease, the question of the practical usage of this knowledge is still open. With current regulations in many countries, academic research groups and private companies cannot share with experiment subjects the information regarding their personal medical risks. That means, that even for those, who could already benefit from the research, the knowledge is inaccessible.

Even more debatable ethical problem is dealing with such risk loci prenatally, using gene editing technics on human embryo. The technique still needs development and the ethical issues still need to be resolved before the actual editing of human genome for pregnancy takes place. Apart for the safety, people also afraid that it will lead to personal traits will be commonly edited. Alas, there is already a screening for the fatal mutations during artificial fertilization, so the more precise editing would be a next logical step.

Alas, the progress cannot be and should not be stopped after all. Any time when new technology emerges, there are doubts and 'end of the world' prophecies, but in several years or decades people cannot imagine the life before the invention. The same is expected from personalized genomics in clinics, when the therapy becomes more available for common patients.

3. CURRENT RESEARCH

The extensive research on 12 major neurological diseases is already taking place. The consortiums, global alliances of laboratories around the world, and government initiatives the large-scale data collection and analysis is now possible. There are several major projects working on connecting genotype and phenotype in neurogenomis: BrainSpan atlas, Psychiatric Genomics Consortium, CommonMind Consortium, The 1000 Genomes Project, Genotype- Tissue Expression program, COCORO, ENCODE and ENIGMA[9].

The databases on disease-related genomes include single nucleotide polymorphisms, copy number variations, insertions and deletions of genes and loss or retention of homozygosity.

For next several decades, brain disorders along with cancer will be a frontier of the personalized medicine developing. With a huge variety, subjective diagnosis and complexity of nature-nuture interactions, it is a challenge for any sole method of discovery, even genomics. Technology itself cannot solve all mentioned problems. Thus, we will need a coordination of researches of different fields. Together neuroscientists, clinicians and bioinformatics have a good chance to prevent, ameliorate and treat the numerous complex neurological diseases triggered by various inherited and environmental causes.

4. FINAL VERDICT

There are many other clinical fields that can benefit from personal genomics studies. As a neurobiologist, I am mostly concerned about neurological and psychiatric diseases. Due to their complexity and pleotropic phenotypes it is almost impossible to find a 'silver bullet' for complex disease.

So, we should approach this matters individually. And of course, everything that is custom

8

made for the persons needs is better than universal, whether it is cloth, software or antipsychotic drug. Though, a strictly personalized approach seems to me overoptimistic. For this we should guarantee equally high standard medical access to all and deal with human conservatism and ignorance, and it could take another millennium to even approach. For now, I think it is reasonable not not to choose between two extremes: tailored medicine and '1 size fits all'[10]. There is always a third compromising option: several standard sizes, which in our case several types of therapy for different types of the same neurological disorder different and patient groups.

REFERENCES

[1]   M. S. Boguski and A. R. Jones, "Neurogenomics: at the intersection of neurobiology and genome sciences.," *Nat. Neurosci.*, vol. 7, no. 5, pp. 429–33, 2004.

[2]   P. M. Thompson, O. A. Andreassen, A. Arias-Vasquez, C. E. Bearden, P. S. Boedhoe, R. M. Brouwer, R. L. Buckner, J. K. Buitelaar, K. B. Bulaeva, D. M. Cannon, R. A. Cohen, P. J. Conrod, A. M. Dale, I. J. Deary, E. L. Dennis, M. A. de Reus, S. Desrivieres, D. Dima, G. Donohoe, S. E. Fisher, J.-P. Fouche, C. Francks, S. Frangou, B. Franke, H. Ganjgahi, H. Garavan, D. C. Glahn, H. J. Grabe, T. Guadalupe, B. A. Gutman, R. Hashimoto, D. P. Hibar, D. Holland, M. Hoogman, H. E. H. Pol, N. Hosten, N. Jahanshad, S. Kelly, P. Kochunov, W. S. Kremen, P. H. Lee, S. Mackey, N. G. Martin, B. Mazoyer, C. McDonald, S. E. Medland, R. A. Morey, T. E. Nichols, T. Paus, Z. Pausova, L. Schmaal, G. Schumann, L. Shen, S. M. Sisodiya, D. J. A. Smit, J. W. Smoller, D. J. Stein, J. L. Stein, R. Toro, J. A. Turner, M. van den Heuvel, O. A. van den Heuvel, T. G. M. van Erp, D. van Rooij, D. J. Veltman, H. Walter, Y. Wang, J. M. Wardlaw, C. D. Whelan, M. J. Wright, and J. Ye, "ENIGMA and the Individual: Predicting Factors that Affect the Brain in 35 Countries Worldwide," *Neuroimage*, 2015.

[3]   J. R. B. Katarzyna Drozda, Daniel J. Müller, "Pharmacogenomic Testing for Neuropsychiatric Drugs: Current Status of Drug Labeling, Guidelines for Using Genetic Information, and Test Options," *Pharmacotherapy.*, no. 4, pp. 166–184, 2014.

[4]   G. L. Cavalleri, M. McCormack, S. Alhusaini, E. Chaila, and N. Delanty, "Pharmacogenomics and epilepsy: the road ahead," *Pharmacogenomics*, vol. 12, no. 10, pp. 1429–1447, 2011.

[5]   L. Spinney, "Alzheimer's disease: The forgetting gene.," *Nature*, vol. 510, no. 7503, pp. 26–8, Jun. 2014.

[6]   B. J. Walters, A. B. Azam, C. J. Gillon, S. A. Josselyn, I. B. Zovkic, and S. A. Josselyn, "Advanced In vivo Use of CRISPR / Cas9 and Anti-sense DNA Inhibition for Gene Manipulation in the Brain," vol. 6, no. January, pp. 1–13, 2016.

[7]   M. Costa-Mattioli and L. M. Monteggia, "mTOR complexes in neurodevelopmental and neuropsychiatric disorders.," *Nat. Neurosci.*, vol. 16, no. 11, pp. 1537–43, Nov. 2013.

[8] G. A. Higgins, A. Allyn-Feuer, S. Handelman, W. Sadee, and B. D. Athey, "The epigenome, 4D nucleome and next-generation neuropsychiatric pharmacogenomics.," *Pharmacogenomics*, vol. 16, no. 14, pp. 1649–69, 2015.

[9] A. C. Mitchell and K. Mirnics, "Gene expression profiling of the brain: Pondering facts and fiction," *Neurobiol. Dis.*, vol. 45, no. 1, pp. 3–7, 2012.

[10] R. I. Horwitz, M. R. Cullen, J. Abell, and J. B. Christian, "(De) Personalized Medicine," vol. 339, no. March, pp. 1155–1157, 2013.

YOUR KNOWLEDGE HAS VALUE

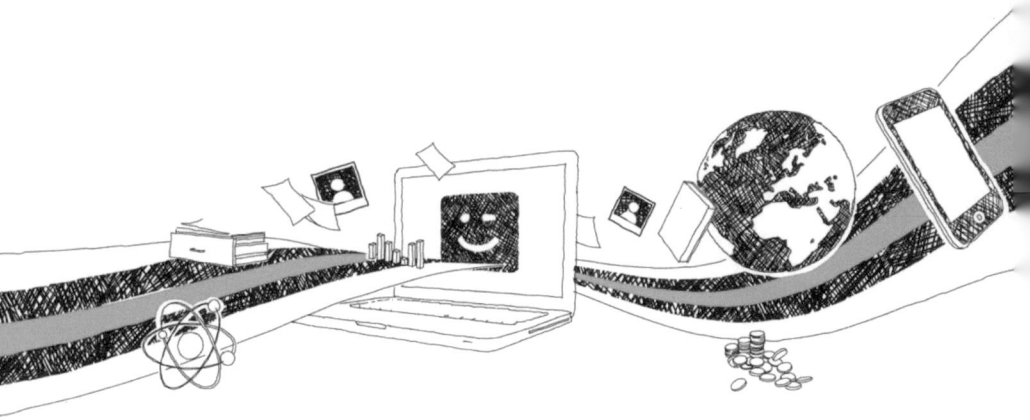

- We will publish your bachelor's and master's thesis, essays and papers

- Your own eBook and book - sold worldwide in all relevant shops

- Earn money with each sale

Upload your text at www.GRIN.com and publish for free

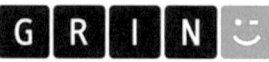